The Complete Lean & Green Breakfast & Lunch Recipe Book

Amazing Lean & Green Breakfast & Lunch Recipes To Lose Weight

Jesse Cohen

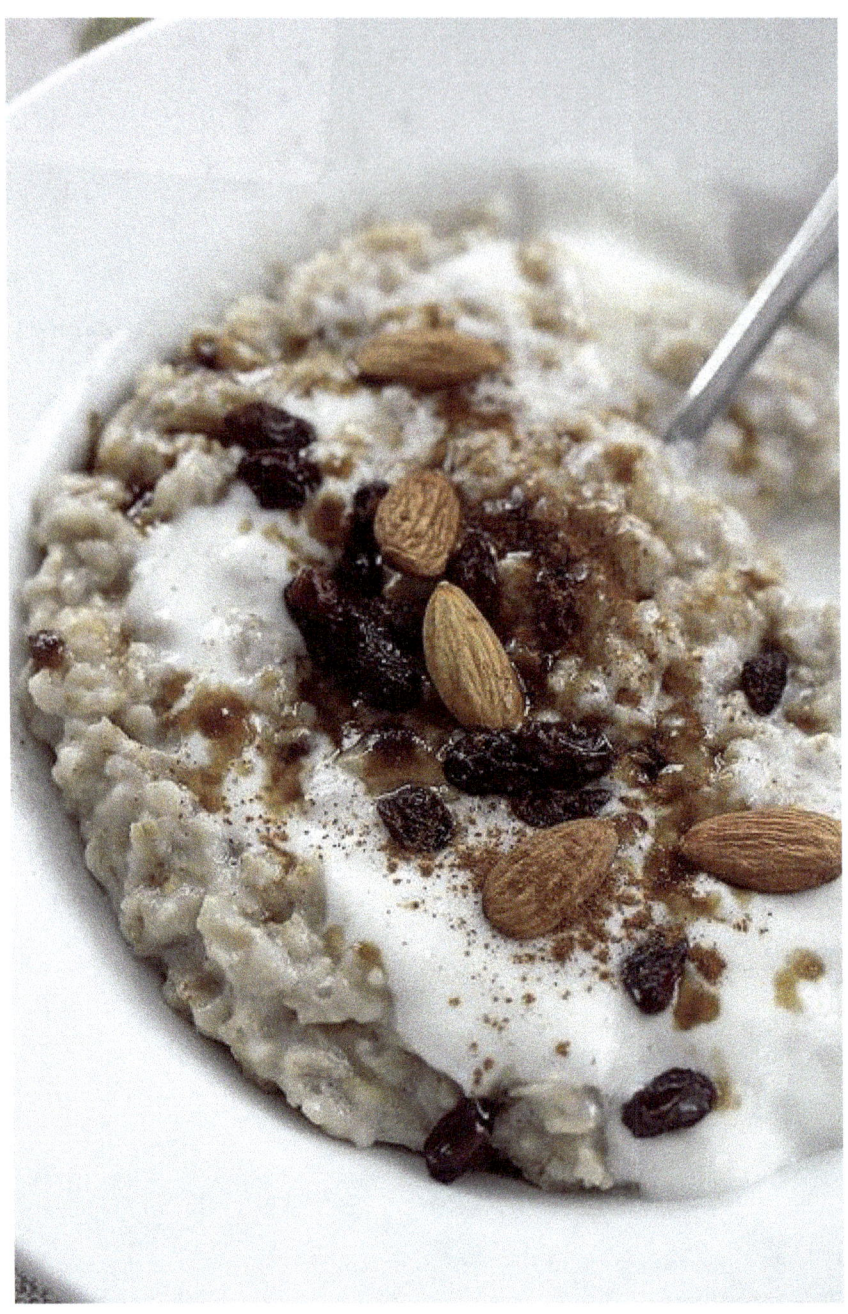

© **Copyright 2020 - All rights reserved.**

The content contained within this book may not be reproduced, duplicated or transmitted without direct written permission from the author or the publisher.

Under no circumstances will any blame or legal responsibility be held against the publisher, or author, for any damages, reparation, or monetary loss due to the information contained within this book. Either directly or indirectly.

Legal Notice:

This book is copyright protected. This book is only for personal use. You cannot amend, distribute, sell, use, quote or paraphrase any part, or the content within this book, without the consent of the author or publisher.

Disclaimer Notice:

Please note the information contained within this document is for educational and entertainment purposes only. All effort has been executed to present accurate, up to date, and reliable, complete information. No warranties of any kind are declared or implied. Readers acknowledge that the author is not engaging in the rendering of legal, financial, medical or professional advice. The content within this book has been derived from various sources. Please consult a licensed professional before attempting any techniques outlined in this book.

By reading this document, the reader agrees that under no circumstances is the author responsible for any losses, direct or indirect, which are incurred as a result of the use of information contained within this document, including, but not limited to, — errors, omissions, or inaccuracies.

Table of contents

Mouth-watering Pie 7

Peanut Butter and Cacao Breakfast Quinoa 9

Chicken Omelet 11

Almond Coconut Cereal 13

WW Salad in a Jar 15

Almond Porridge 17

Special Almond Cereal 19

Bacon and Lemon spiced Muffins 21

Vitamin C Smoothie Cubes 23

Greek Style Mini Burger Pies 25

Awesome Avocado Muffins 27

Raw-Cinnamon-Apple Nut Bowl 29

Family Fun Pizza 31

Tasty WW Pancakes 34

Slow Cooker Savory Butternut Squash Oatmeal 36

Yummy Smoked Salmon 38

Spiced Sorghum and Berries 40

WW Breakfast Cereal 42

Asparagus Frittata Recipe 44

Avocados Stuffed with Salmon 46

Tropical Greens Smoothie 48

Overnight Chocolate Chia Pudding 50

Carrot Cake Oatmeal 52

Bacon Spaghetti Squash Carbonara 54

Vanilla Buckwheat Porridge 56

Cauliflower Rice 58

Jarlsberg Lunch Omelet 60

Stuffed Mushrooms 62

Jalapeno Cheese Balls 64

Zucchini Omelet 67

Courgette Risotto 69

Cheesy Cauliflower Fritters 71

Bell-Pepper Corn Wrapped in Tortilla 73

Zucchini Parmesan Chips 75

Prosciutto Spinach Salad 77

Crispy Roasted Broccoli 79

Grilled Ham & Cheese 81

Coconut Battered Cauliflower Bites 83

Mashed Garlic Turnips 85

Air Fryer Asparagus 87

Diced Cauliflower & Curry Chicken 89

Jalapeno Coins 91

Lasagna Spaghetti Squash 93

Monkey Salad 95

Mu Shu Lunch Pork 97

Fiery Jalapeno Poppers 99

Bacon & Chicken Patties...101

Garlic Chicken Balls..103

Cheddar Bacon Burst..105

Blue Cheese Chicken Wedges...107

Mouth-watering Pie

Preparation Time: 15 minutes

Cooking Time: 45 minutes

Servings: 8

Ingredients:

- 3/4-pound of beef; ground
- 1/2 onion; chopped.
- 1 pie crust
- 3 tablespoons of taco seasoning
- 1 teaspoon of baking soda
- Mango salsa for serving
- 1/2 red bell pepper; chopped.
- A handful cilantro; chopped.
- 8 eggs
- 1 teaspoon of coconut oil
- Salt and black pepper to the taste.

Directions:

1. Heat up a pan, add oil, beef, cook until it browns and mix with salt, pepper, and taco seasoning.
2. Stir again, transfer to a bowl and leave aside for now.
3. Heat up the pan again over medium heat with cooking juices from the meat, add onion and pepper; stir and cook for 4 minutes
4. Add eggs, baking soda and a few salt and stir well.
5. Add cilantro; stir again and start heating.
6. Spread beef mix in pie shell, add veggies mix and cover meat, heat oven at 350° F and bake for 45 minutes.
7. Leave the pie to chill down a bit, slice, divide between plates and serve with mango salsa on top.

Nutrition:

- Calories: 198
- Fat: 11 g
- Fiber: 1 g
- Carbs: 12 g
- Protein: 12 g

Peanut Butter and Cacao Breakfast Quinoa

Preparation Time: 5 Minutes

Cooking Time: 10 Minutes

Servings: 1

Ingredients:

- 1/3 cup of quinoa flakes
- 1/2 cup of unsweetened nondairy milk,
- 1/2 cup of water
- 1/8 cup of raw cacao powder
- One tablespoon of natural creamy peanut butter
- 1/8 teaspoon of ground cinnamon
- One banana; mashed
- Fresh berries of choice; for serving
- Chopped nuts of choice; for serving

Directions:

- Using an 8-quart pot over medium-high heat, mix together the quinoa flakes, milk, water, cacao powder, spread, and cinnamon.
- Cook and stir it until the mixture begins to simmer. Turn the heat to medium-low and cook for 3-5 minutes, stirring frequently.
- Stir in the bananas and cook until hot.
- Serve topped with fresh berries, nuts, and a splash of milk.

Nutrition:
- Calories: 471
- Fat: 16 g
- Protein: 18 g
- Carbohydrates: 69 g
- Fiber: 16 g

Chicken Omelet

Preparation Time: 5 minutes

Cooking Time: 15 minutes

Servings: 1

Ingredients:

- 2 bacon slices; cooked and crumbled
- 2 eggs
- 1 tablespoon of homemade mayonnaise
- 1 tomato; chopped.
- 1-ounce of rotisserie chicken; shredded
- 1 teaspoon of mustard
- 1 small avocado; pitted, peeled and chopped.
- Salt and black pepper to the taste.

Directions:

1. In a bowl, mix eggs with some salt and pepper and whisk gently.
2. Heat up a pan over medium heat, spray with some vegetable oil, add eggs and cook your omelet for 5 minutes.

Add chicken, avocado, tomato, bacon, mayo and mustard on one half of the omelet.
3. Fold omelet, cover pan and cook for 5 minutes more.
4. Transfer to a plate and serve.

Nutrition:

- Calories: 400
- Fat: 32 g
- Fiber: 6 g
- Carbs: 4 g
- Protein: 25 g

Almond Coconut Cereal

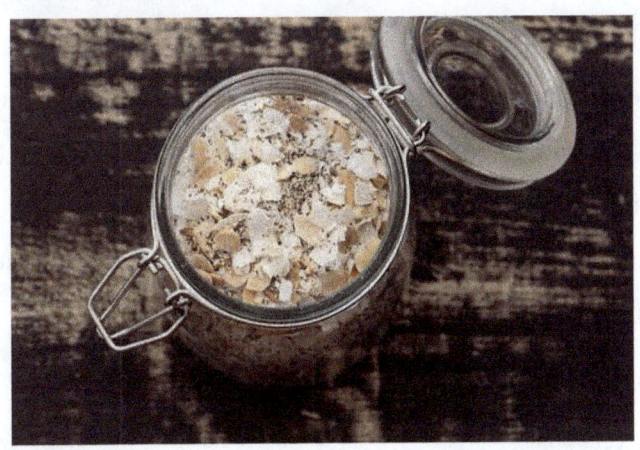

Preparation Time: 5 minutes

Cooking Time: 5 minutes

Servings: 2

Ingredients:

- 1/3 cup of Water.
- 1/3 cup of Coconut milk.
- 2 tbsps. of Roasted sunflower seeds.
- 1 tbsp. of Chia seeds.
- ½ cup of Blueberries.
- 2 tbsps. of Chopped almonds.

Directions:

1. Put a medium bowl in position and add coconut milk and chia seeds, then put aside for 5 minutes.
2. Blend almond with sunflower seeds, then add the mixture to the chia seeds mixture and add water to make them mix evenly.
3. Serve topped with the remaining sunflower seeds and blueberries.

Nutrition:

- Calories: 181
- Fat: 15.2 g
- Fiber: 4 g
- Carbs: 10.8 g
- Protein: 3.7 g

WW Salad in a Jar

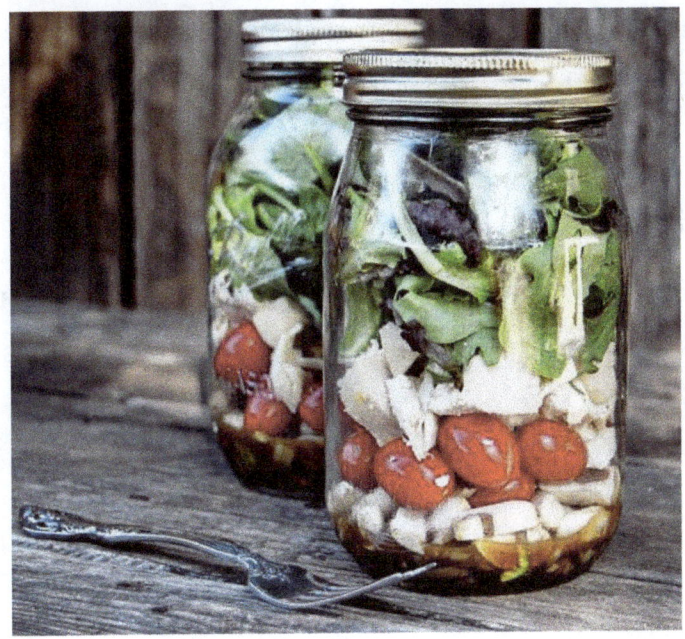

Preparation Time: 10 minutes

Cooking Time: 5 minutes

Servings: 1

Ingredients:

- 1-ounce of favorite greens
- 1-ounce of red bell pepper; chopped.
- 4 ounces' of rotisserie chicken; roughly chopped.
- 4 tablespoons of extra virgin olive oil

- 1/2 scallion; chopped.
- 1-ounce of cucumber; chopped.
- 1-ounce of cherry tomatoes; halved
- Salt and black pepper to taste.

Directions:

1. In a bowl, mix greens with red bell pepper, tomatoes, scallion, cucumber, salt, pepper, olive oil, and toss to coat well.
2. Transfer this to a jar, top with chicken pieces and serve for breakfast.

Nutrition:

- Calories: 180
- Fat: 12 g
- Fiber: 4 g
- Carbs: 5 g
- Protein: 17 g

Almond Porridge

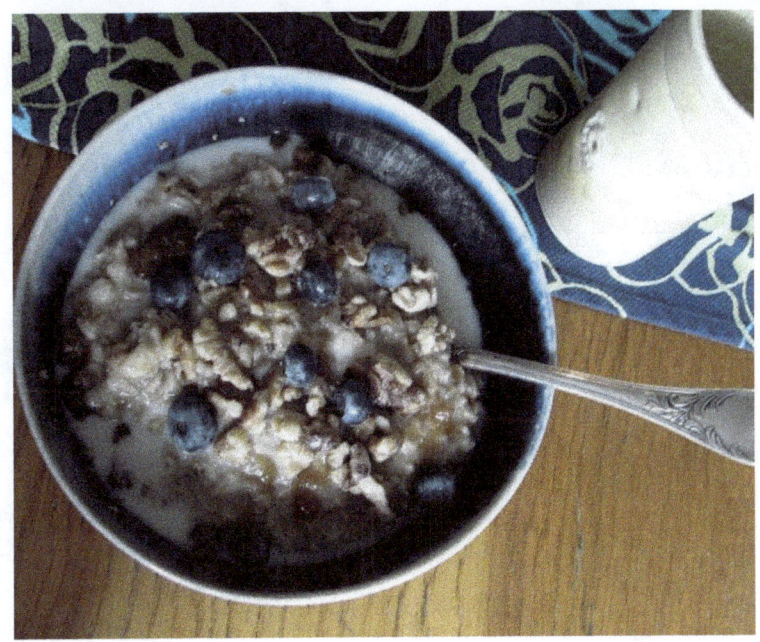

Preparation Time: 10 minutes

Cooking Time: 5 minutes

Servings: 1

Ingredients:

- ¼ tsp. of Ground cloves.
- ¼ tsp. of Nutmeg.
- 1 tsp. of Stevia.
- ¾ cup of Coconut cream.

- ½ cup of Ground almonds.
- ¼ tsp. of Ground cardamom.
- 1 tsp. of Ground cinnamon.

Directions:

1. Set your pan over medium heat to cook the coconut milk for a couple of minutes
2. Stir in almonds and stevia to cook for 5 minutes
3. Mix in nutmeg, cardamom, and cinnamon.
4. Enjoy while still hot.

Nutrition:

- Calories: 695
- Fat: 66.7 g
- Fiber: 11.1 g
- Carbs: 22 g
- Protein: 14.3 g

Special Almond Cereal

Preparation Time: 5 minutes

Cooking Time: 5 minutes

Servings: 1

Ingredients:

- 2 tablespoons of almonds; chopped.
- 1/3 cup of coconut milk
- 1 tablespoon of chia seeds
- 2 tablespoon of pepitas; roasted
- A handful blueberries
- 1 small banana; chopped.
- 1/3 cup of water

1. **Directions:**
2. In a bowl, mix chia seeds with coconut milk and leave aside for 5 minutes. In your food processor, mix half the pepitas with almonds and pulse them well.
3. Add this to chia seeds mix.

4. Also add the water and stir.
5. Top with the rest of the pepitas, banana pieces, blueberries, and serve.

Nutrition:

- Calories: 200
- Fat: 3 g
- Fiber: 2 g
- Carbs: 5 g
- Protein: 4 g

Bacon and Lemon spiced Muffins

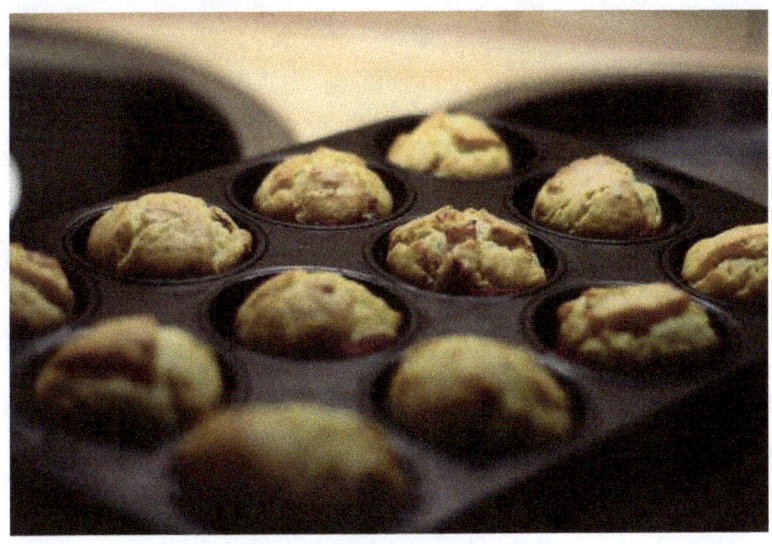

Preparation Time: 10 minutes

Cooking Time: 20 minutes

Servings: 12

Ingredients:

- 2 tsps. of Lemon thyme.
- Salt
- 3 cup of Almond flour.
- ½ cup of Melted butter.
- 1 tsp. of Baking soda.

- Black pepper
- 1 cup of Medium eggs.
- 4 Diced bacon.

Directions:

1. Set a bowl in place and mix the eggs and baking soda very well. Whisk in the seasonings, butter, bacon, and lemon thyme. Set the mixture in a well-lined muffin pan.
2. Set the oven for 20 minutes at 350º F, and allow to bake.
3. Allow the muffins to chill before serving.

Nutrition:

- Calories: 186
- Fat: 17.1 g
- Fiber: 0.8 g
- Carbs: 1.8 g
- Protein: 7.4 g

Vitamin C Smoothie Cubes

Preparation Time: 5 minutes

Cooking Time: 8 hours to chill

Servings: 1

Ingredients:

- 1/8 large papaya
- 1/8 mango
- 1/4 cups of chopped pineapple; fresh or frozen
- 1/8 cup of raw cauliflower florets; fresh or frozen
- 1/4 large navel oranges; peeled and halved
- 1/4 large orange bell pepper stemmed, seeded, and coarsely chopped

Directions:

1. Halve the papaya and mango, remove the pits, and scoop their soft flesh into a high-speed blender.
2. Add the pineapple, cauliflower, oranges, and bell pepper. Blend until smooth.

3. Evenly divide the puree between 2 (16-compartment) cube trays and place them on a level surface in your freezer. Freeze for a minimum of 8 hours.
4. The cubes are often left in the cube trays until use or transferred to a freezer bag. The frozen cubes are good for about three weeks in a standard freezer, or up to six months in a chest freezer.

Nutrition:
- Calories: 96
- Fat: 1 g
- Protein: 2 g
- Carbohydrates: 24 g
- Fiber: 4 g

Greek Style Mini Burger Pies

Preparation Time: 15 minutes

Cooking Time: 40 minutes

Servings: 6

Ingredients:

Burger mixture:

- Onion, large, chopped (1 piece)
- Red bell peppers, roasted, diced (1/2 cup)
- Ground lamb, 80% lean (1 pound)
- Red pepper flakes (1/4 teaspoon) Feta cheese, crumbled (2 ounces)

Baking mixture:

- Milk (1/2 cup)
- Biscuit mix, classic (1/2 cup)
- Eggs (2 pieces)

Directions:

1. Preheat oven at 350º F.
2. Grease 12 muffin cups using cooking spray.

3. Cook the onion and beef in a skillet heated on medium-high. Once beef is browned and cooked through, drain and allow to cool for 5 minutes. Stir with feta cheese, roasted red peppers, and red pepper flakes.
4. Whisk the baking mixture ingredients together. Fill each muffin cup with baking mixture (1 tablespoon).
5. Air-fry for twenty-five to thirty minutes. Let cool before serving.

Nutrition:

- Calories 270
- Fat: 10 g
- Protein: 10 g
- Carbohydrates: 10 g

Awesome Avocado Muffins

Preparation Time: 10 minutes

Cooking Time: 20 minutes

Servings: 12

Ingredients:

- 6 bacon slices; chopped.
- 1 yellow onion; chopped.
- 1/2 teaspoon of baking soda
- 1/2 cup of coconut flour
- 1 cup of coconut milk
- 2 cups of avocado; pitted, peeled and chopped.
- 4 eggs
- Salt and black pepper to taste.

Directions:

1. Heat up a pan, add onion and bacon; stir and brown for a couple of minutes. In a bowl, mash avocado pieces with a fork and whisk well with the eggs. Add milk, salt, pepper, baking soda, coconut flour, and stir everything.

2. Add bacon mix and stir again.
3. Add coconut oil to muffin tray, divide eggs and avocado mix into the tray, heat oven at 350º F and bake for 20 minutes
4. Divide muffins between plates and serve them for breakfast.

Nutrition:
- Calories: 200
- Fat: 7 g
- Fiber: 4 g
- Carbs: 7 g
- Protein: 5 g

Raw-Cinnamon-Apple Nut Bowl

Preparation Time: 15 minutes

Cooking Time: 1 hour to chill

Servings: 1

Ingredients:

- One green apple; halved, seeded, and cored
- 3/4 Honeycrisp apples; halved, seeded, and cored
- 1/4 teaspoon of freshly squeezed lemon juice
- One pitted Medrol dates
- 1/8 teaspoon of ground cinnamon
- Pinch of ground nutmeg
- 1/2 tablespoons of chia seeds, plus more for serving (optional)
- 1/4 tablespoon of hemp seed
- 1/8 cup of chopped walnuts
- Nut butter, for serving (optional)

Directions:

1. Finely dice half the green apple and one candy apple. Mix with the lemon juice and store in an airtight container while you are executing subsequent steps.
2. Coarsely chop the remaining apples and the dates. Transfer to a food processor and add the cinnamon and nutmeg.
3. Check it several times to see if it's mixing, then process for 2 to 3 minutes to puree. Stir the puree into the reserved diced apples.
4. Stir in the chia seeds (if using), hemp seeds, and walnuts.
5. Chill for a minimum of one hour.
6. Enjoy!
7. Serve as it is or top with additional chia seeds and spread (if using).

Nutrition:

- Calories: 274
- Fat: 8 g
- Protein: 4 g
- Carbohydrates: 52 g
- Fiber: 9 g

Family Fun Pizza

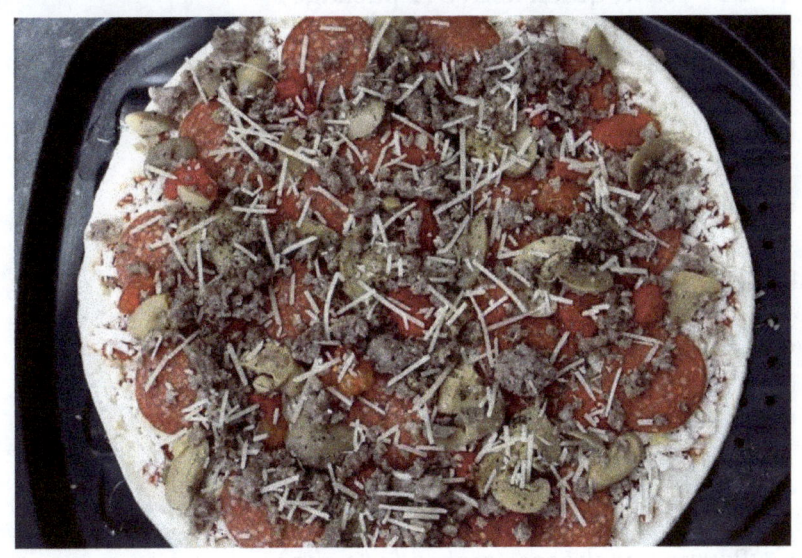

Preparation Time: 30 minutes

Cooking Time: 25 minutes

Servings: 16

Ingredients:

Pizza crust:

- Water; warm (1 cup)
- Salt (1/2 teaspoon)
- Flour, whole wheat (1 cup)

- Olive oil (2 tablespoons)
- Dry yeast; quick active (1 package)
- Flour, all purpose (1 ½ cups)
- Cornmeal
- Olive oil

Filling:

- Onion; chopped (1 cup)
- Mushrooms; sliced, drained (4 ounces)
- Garlic cloves; chopped finely (2 pieces)
- Parmesan cheese; grated (1/4 cup)
- Ground lamb; 80% lean (1 pound)
- Italian seasoning (1 teaspoon)
- Pizza sauce (8 ounces)
- Mozzarella cheese; shredded (2 cups)

Directions:

1. Mix yeast with warm water. Combine with flours, oil (2 tablespoons), and salt by stirring then beating vigorously for half a minute. Let the dough sit for twenty minutes.
2. Preheat oven at 350° F.

3. Prep 2 square pans (8-inch) by greasing with oil and then sprinkling with cornmeal.
4. Cut the rested dough in half; place each half inside each pan. Set aside, covered, for 30 to 45 minutes. Cook in the airfryer for 20 to 22 minutes.
5. Sauté the onion, beef, garlic, and Italian seasoning until beef is totally cooked. Drain and put aside.
6. Cover the air-fried crusts with pizza sauce before topping with beef mixture, cheeses, and mushrooms.
7. Return to oven and cook for 20 minutes.

Nutrition:
- Calories 215
- Fat 0 g
- Protein 10 g
- Carbohydrates 20.0 g

Tasty WW Pancakes

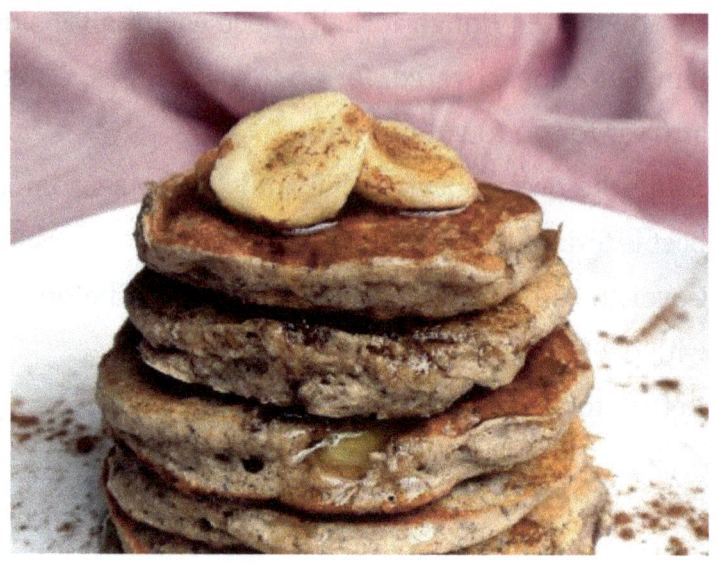

Preparation Time: 12 minutes

Cooking Time: 3 minutes

Servings: 4

Ingredients:

- 2 ounces of cream cheese
- 1 teaspoon of stevia
- 1/2 teaspoon of cinnamon; ground
- 2 eggs
- Cooking spray

Directions:

1. Mix the eggs with the cream cheese, stevia, and cinnamon in a blender, and blend well.
2. Heat pan with cooking spray over medium-high heat. Add 1/4 of the batter, spread well, cook for 2 minutes, invert and cook for 1 minute more.
3. Move to a plate and repeat the process with the rest of the dough.
4. Serve them directly.

Nutrition:

- Calories: 344
- Fat: 23 g
- Fiber: 12 g
- Carbs: 3 g
- Protein: 16 g

Slow Cooker Savory Butternut Squash Oatmeal

Preparation Time: 15 minutes

Cooking Time: 6 to 8 hours

Servings: 1

Ingredients:

- 1/4 cup of steel-cut oats
- 1/2 cups of cubed (1/2-inch pieces), peeled butternut squash (after preparing a whole squash, freeze any leftovers for future meals)
- 3/4 cups of water
- 1/16 cup of unsweetened nondairy milk
- 1/4 tablespoon of chia seeds
- 1/2 teaspoons of yellow miso paste
- 3/4 teaspoons of ground ginger
- 1/4 tablespoon of sesame seeds; toasted
- 1/4 tablespoon of chopped scallion; green parts only
- Shredded carrot, for serving (optional)

Directions:

1. In a slow cooker, mix the oats, butternut squash, and water.
2. Cover the slow cooker and cook on low for 6 to 8 hours, or until the squash is fork-tender.
3. Using a potato masher or heavy spoon, roughly mash the cooked butternut squash.
4. Stir to mix with the oats.
5. Whisk together the milk, chia seeds, miso paste, and ginger in a large bowl. Stir the mixture into the oats.
6. Top your oatmeal bowl with sesame seeds and scallion for more plant-based fiber, and top with shredded carrot (if using).

Nutrition:

- Calories: 230
- Fat: 5 g
- Protein: 7 g
- Carbohydrates: 40 g
- Fiber: 9 g

Yummy Smoked Salmon

Preparation Time: 10 minutes

Cooking Time: 10 minutes

Servings: 3

Ingredients:

- 4 eggs; whisked
- 1/2 teaspoon of avocado oil
- 4 ounces of smoked salmon; chopped.

For the sauce:

- 1/2 cup of cashews; soaked and drained
- 1/4 cup of green onions; chopped.
- 1 teaspoon of garlic powder
- 1 cup of coconut milk
- 1 tablespoon of lemon juice
- Salt and black pepper to taste.

Directions:

1. In your blender, mix cashews with coconut milk, garlic powder, juice, and blend well.

2. Add salt, pepper, green onions, and blend well again. Transfer to a bowl and keep in the fridge for now. Heat up a pan with the oil over medium-low heat; add eggs, whisk a touch and cook until it is almost done. Pour in your preheated broiler and cook until eggs set.
3. Divide eggs on plates, top with salmon and serve with the scallion sauce on top.

Nutrition:

- Calories: 200
- Fat: 10 g
- Fiber: 2 g
- Carbs: 11 g
- Protein: 15 g

Spiced Sorghum and Berries

Preparation Time: 5 minutes

Cooking Time: 1 hour

Servings: 1

Ingredients:

- 1/4 cup of whole-grain sorghum
- 1/4 teaspoon of ground cinnamon
- 1/4 teaspoon of Chinese five-spice powder
- 3/4 cups of water
- 1/4 cup of unsweetened nondairy milk
- 1/4 teaspoon of vanilla extract
- 1/2 tablespoons of pure maple syrup
- 1/2 tablespoon of chia seed
- 1/8 cup of sliced almonds
- 1/2 cups of fresh raspberries; divided

Directions:

1. Place a large pot over medium-high heat, stir in together the sorghum, cinnamon, five-spice powder, and water.
2. Wait for the water to boil, cover it, and reduce the heat to medium-low.
3. Cook for 1 hour, or until the sorghum is soft and chewy. If the sorghum grains are still hard, add another cup of water and cook for 15 minutes more.
4. Using a glass cup, whisk together the milk, vanilla, and syrup to blend.
5. Add the mixture to the sorghum and the chia seeds, almonds, and 1 cup of raspberries. Gently stir to mix.
6. When serving, top with the remaining one cup of fresh raspberries.

Nutrition:

- Calories: 289
- Fat: 8 g
- Protein: 9 g
- Carbohydrates: 52 g
- Fiber: 10 g

WW Breakfast Cereal

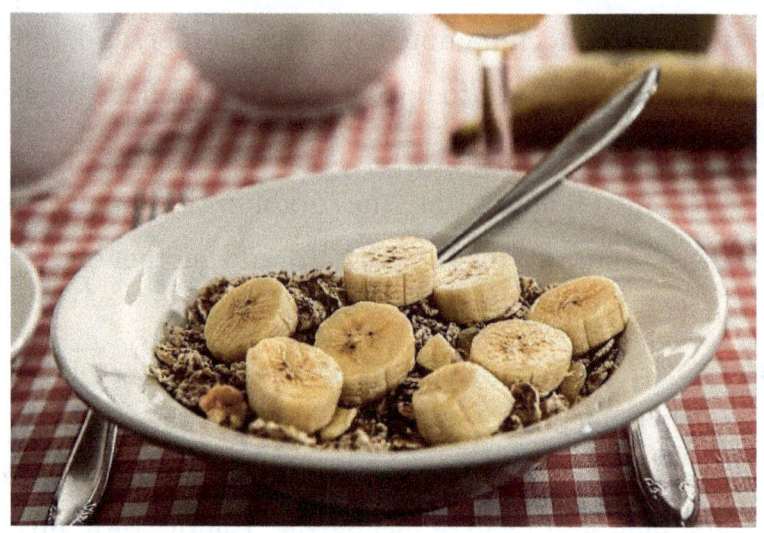

Preparation Time: 10 minutes

Cooking Time: 3 minutes

Servings: 2

Ingredients:

- 1/2 cup of coconut; shredded
- 1/3 cup of macadamia nuts; chopped.
- 4 teaspoons of ghee
- 2 cups of almond milk
- 1 tablespoon of stevia
- 1/3 cup of walnuts; chopped

- 1/3 cup of flax seed
- A pinch of salt

Directions:

1. Heat a pot of mistletoe over medium heat. Add the milk, coconut, salt, macadamia nuts, walnuts, flax seeds, stevia, and blend well.
2. Cook for 3 minutes. Stir again, and remove from heat for 10 minutes.
3. Divide into 2 bowls and serve

Nutrition:

- Calories: 140
- Fat: 3 g
- Fiber: 2 g
- Carbs: 1. 5 g
- Protein: 7 g

Asparagus Frittata Recipe

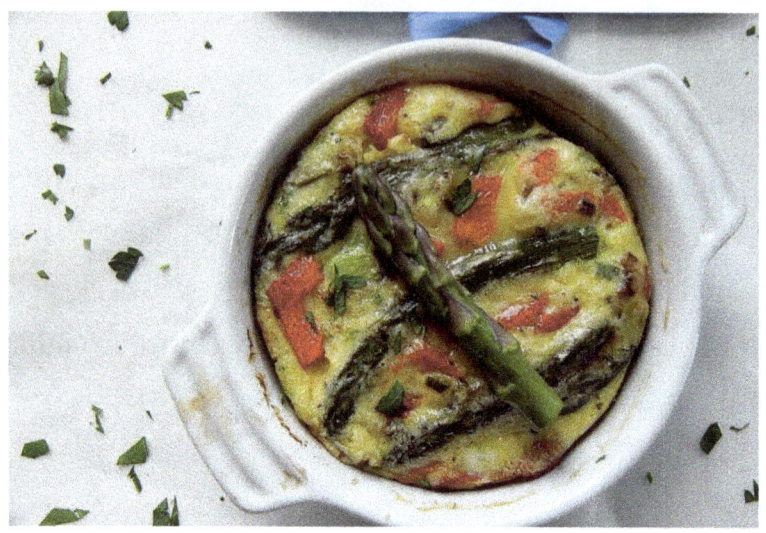

Preparation Time: 20 minutes

Cooking Time: 20 minutes

Servings: 4

Ingredients:

- 4 Bacon slices; chopped
- Salt and black pepper
- 8 Eggs; whisked
- 1 bunch of asparagus; trimmed and chopped

Directions:

1. Heat a pan, add bacon, stir and cook for 5 minutes.
2. Add asparagus, salt, and pepper, stir and cook for an additional 5 minutes.
3. Add the chilled eggs, spread them in the pan, allow them to substitute the oven and bake for 20 minutes at 350°F.
4. Share and divide between plates and serve for breakfast.

Nutrition:

- Calories: 251
- Carbs: 16 g
- Fat: 6 g
- Fiber: 8 g
- Protein: 7 g

Avocados Stuffed with Salmon

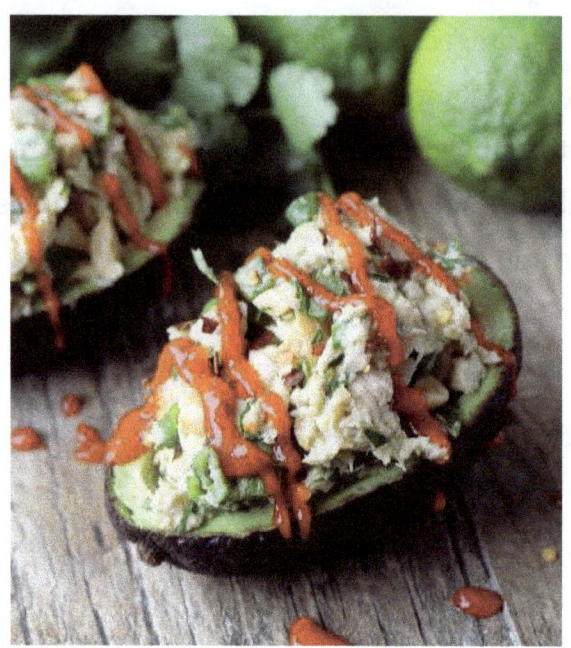

Preparation Time: 5 minutes

Cooking Time: 5 minutes

Servings: 2

Ingredients:

- 1 Avocado; pitted and halved
- 2 tablespoons of olive oil
- 1 Lemon juice
- 2 ounces of Smoked salmon; flaked

- 1 ounce of Goat cheese; crumbled
- Salt and black pepper

Directions:

1. Mix the salmon with lemon juice, olive oil, cheese, salt, and pepper in your food processor and pulsate well.
2. Divide this mixture into avocado halves and serve.
3. Dish and Enjoy!

Nutrition:

- Calories: 300
- Fat: 15 g
- Fiber: 5 g
- Carbs: 8 g
- Protein: 16 g

Tropical Greens Smoothie

Preparation Time: 5 Minutes

Cooking Time: 0 Minutes

Servings: 1

Ingredients:

- 1 banana
- 1/2 large navel orange; peeled and segmented
- 1/2 cup of frozen mango chunks
- 1 cup of frozen spinach
- 1 celery stalk; broken into pieces
- 1 tablespoon of cashew butter or almond butter
- 1/2 tablespoon of spiraling
- 1/2 tablespoon of ground flaxseed
- 1/2 cup of unsweetened nondairy milk
- Water; for thinning (optional)

Directions:

1. In a high-speed blender or food processor, mix the bananas, orange, mango, spinach, celery, cashew butter, spiraling (if using), flaxseed, and milk.

2. Blend until creamy, adding more milk or water to thin the smoothie if too thick. Serve immediately—it is best served fresh.

Nutrition:

- Calories: 391
- Fat: 12 g
- Protein: 13 g
- Carbohydrates: 68 g
- Fiber: 13 g

Overnight Chocolate Chia Pudding

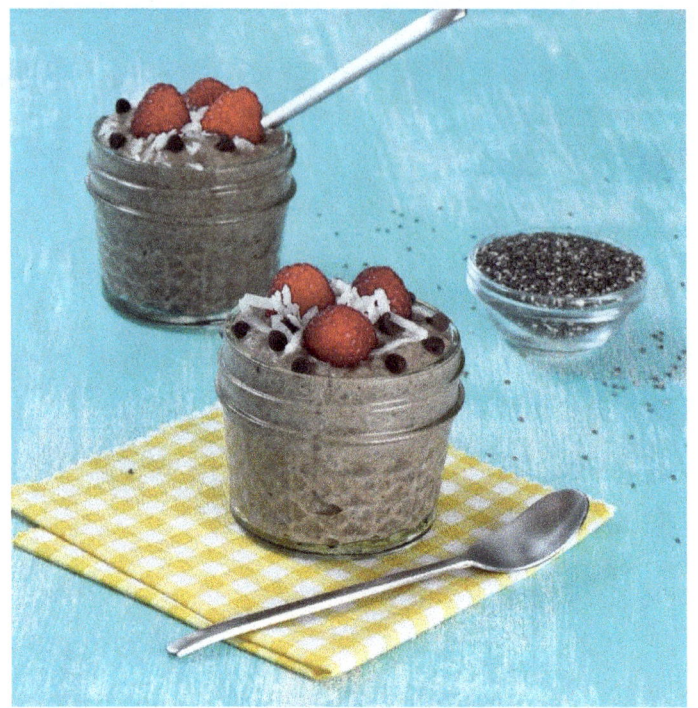

Preparation Time: 2 minutes

Cooking Time: overnight to chill

Servings: 1

Ingredients:

- 1/8 cup of chia seeds
- 1/2 cup of unsweetened nondairy milk

- 1 tablespoon of raw cocoa powder
- 1/2 teaspoon of vanilla extract
- 1/2 teaspoon of pure maple syrup

Directions:

1. Mix together the chia seeds, milk, cacao powder, vanilla, and syrup in a large bowl.
2. Divide between two (1/2-pint) covered glass jars or containers.
3. Refrigerate overnight.
4. Stir before serving.

Nutrition:

- Calories: 213
- Fat: 10 g
- Protein: 9 g
- Carbohydrates: 20 g
- Fiber: 15 g

Carrot Cake Oatmeal

Preparation Time: 10 minutes

Cooking Time: 15 minutes

Servings: 1

Ingredients:

- 1/8 cup of pecans
- 1/2 cup of finely shredded carrot
- 1/4 cup of old-fashioned oats
- 5/8 cups of unsweetened nondairy milk
- 1/2 tablespoon of pure maple syrup
- 1/2 teaspoon of ground cinnamon
- 1/2 teaspoon of ground ginger
- 1/8 teaspoon of ground nutmeg
- 1 tablespoon of chia seed

Directions:

1. Over medium-high heat in a skillet, toast the pecans for 3 to 4 minutes, often stirring, until browned and fragrant (watch closely, as they will burn quickly).

2. Pour the pecans onto a chopping board and coarsely chop them. Set aside.
3. In an 8-quart pot over medium-high heat, mix the carrot, oats, milk, maple syrup, cinnamon, ginger, and nutmeg.
4. When it has started boiling, reduce the heat to medium-low.
5. Cook, uncovered, for 10 minutes, stirring occasionally.
6. Stir in the chopped pecans and chia seeds. Serve immediately.

Nutrition:

- Calories: 307
- Fat: 17 g
- Protein: 7 g
- Carbohydrates: 35 g
- Fiber: 11 g

Bacon Spaghetti Squash Carbonara

Preparation Time: 20 minutes

Cooking Time: 40 minutes

Servings: 4

Ingredients:

- 1 small spaghetti squash
- 6 ounces of bacon (roughly chopped)
- 1 large tomato; sliced
- 2 chives; chopped
- 1 garlic clove; minced
- 6 ounces of low-fat cottage cheese
- 1 cup of Gouda cheese; grated
- 2 tablespoons of olive oil
- Salt and pepper, to taste

Directions:

1. Preheat the oven to 350°F.
2. Cut the squash spaghetti in half, brush with some vegetable oil and bake for 20–30 minutes, skin side up.

Remove from the oven and take away the core with a fork, creating the spaghetti.

3. Heat one tablespoon of olive oil in a skillet. Cook the bacon for about 1 minute until crispy.
4. Quickly wipe out the pan with paper towels.
5. Heat another tablespoon of oil and sauté the garlic, tomato, and chives for 2–3 minutes. Add the spaghetti and sauté for an additional 5 minutes, occasionally stirring to keep from burning.
6. Start putting in the pot cheese, about 2 tablespoons at a time. If the sauce becomes thick, add a few cups of water. The sauce should be creamy but not too runny or thick. Allow to cook for an additional 3 minutes.
7. Serve immediately.

Nutrition:

- Calories: 305
- Total Fat: 21 g
- Net Carbs: 8 g
- Protein: 18 g

Vanilla Buckwheat Porridge

Preparation Time: 5 minutes

Cooking Time: 25 minutes

Servings: 1

Ingredients:

- 1 cup of water
- 1/4 cup of raw buckwheat grouts
- 1/4 teaspoon of ground cinnamon
- 1/4 banana; sliced
- 1/16 cup of golden raisins
- 1/16 cup of dried currants
- 1/16 cup of sunflower seeds
- 1/2 tablespoons of chia seeds
- 1/4 tablespoon of hemp seeds
- 1/4 tablespoon of sesame seeds, toasted
- 1/8 cup of unsweetened nondairy milk
- 1/4 tablespoon of pure maple syrup
- 1/4 teaspoon of vanilla extract

Directions:

1. Boil the water in a pot. Stir in the buckwheat, cinnamon, and banana.
2. Cook the mixture and wait for it to boil, then reduce the heat to medium-low.
3. Cover the pot and cook for 15 minutes, or until the buckwheat is soft and then remove from the heat.
4. Stir in the raisins, currants, sunflower seeds, chia seeds, hemp seeds, sesame seeds, milk, maple syrup, and vanilla. Cover the pot. Wait for 10 minutes before serving.
5. Serve as it is or top as desired.

Nutrition:

- Calories: 353
- Fat: 11 g
- Protein: 10 g
- Carbohydrates: 61 g
- Fiber: 10 g

Cauliflower Rice

Preparation Time: 5 minutes

Cooking Time: 20 minutes

Servings: 1

Ingredients:

Round 1:

- 1/2 tsp. of turmeric
- 1/2 cup of diced carrot
- 1/8 cup of diced onion
- 1/2 tbsp. of low-sodium soy sauce
- 1/8 block of extra firm tofu

Round 2:

- 1/2 cup of frozen peas
- 1/4 minced garlic cloves
- 1/2 cup of chopped broccoli
- 1/2 tbsp. of minced ginger
- 1/4 tbsp. of rice vinegar
- 1/4 tsp. of toasted sesame oil

- 1/2 tbsp. of reduced-sodium soy sauce
- 1/2 cup of diced cauliflower

Directions:

1. Crush tofu in a large bowl and toss with all the Round one ingredient.
2. Lock the air fryer lid—preheat the instant crisp airfryer to 370° F. Also, set the temperature to 370°F, set time to 10 minutes, and cook for 10 minutes, making sure to shake once.
3. In another bowl, toss ingredients from Round 2 together.
4. Add Round 2 mixture to instant crisp airfryer and cook for another 5 to 10 minutes.
5. Enjoy!

Nutrition:

- Calories: 67
- Fat: 8 g
- Protein: 3 g
- Sugar: 0 g

Jarlsberg Lunch Omelet

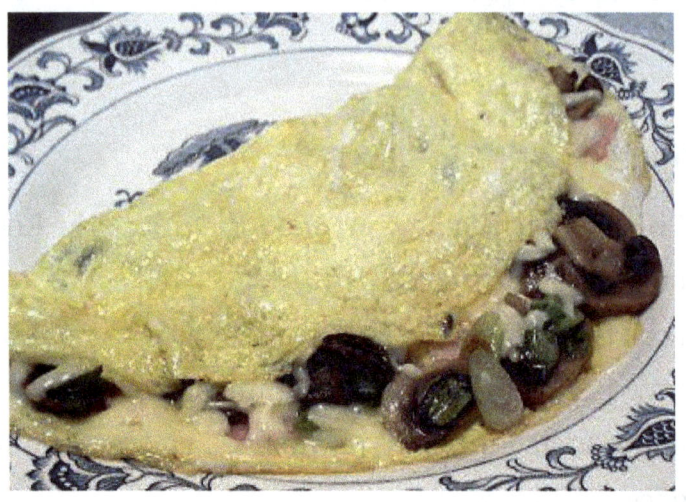

Preparation Time: 5 minutes

Cooking Time: 10 minutes

Servings: 2

Ingredients:

- 4 medium mushrooms; sliced, 2 oz.
- 1 green onion; sliced
- 2 eggs; beaten
- 1 oz. of Jarlsberg or Swiss cheese; shredded
- 1 oz. of ham; diced

Directions:

1. In a skillet, cook the mushrooms and scallion until soft.
2. Add the eggs and blend well.
3. Sprinkle with salt and top with the mushroom mixture, cheese, and the ham.
4. When the egg is settled, fold the plain side of the omelet on the filled side.
5. Turn off the heat and let it stand until the cheese has melted.
6. Serve!

Nutrition:

- Calories: 288
- Carbs: 22 g
- Fat: 12 g
- Protein: 27 g
- Fiber: 6 g

Stuffed Mushrooms

Preparation Time: 7 minutes

Cooking Time: 8 minutes

Servings: 1

Ingredients:

- 1/2 rashers bacon; diced
- 1/2 onion; diced
- 1/2 bell pepper; diced
- 1/2 small carrot; diced
- 2 medium size mushrooms (separate the caps and stalks)
- 1/4 cup of shredded cheddar plus extra for two top
- 1/4 cup of sour cream

Directions:

1. Chop the mushrooms stalks finely and fry them up with the bacon, onion, pepper, and carrot at 350°F for 8 minutes.

2. Also, check when the veggies are soft, and stir in the soured cream and the cheese. Keep up the heat until the cheese has melted, and everything is mixed nicely.
3. Now grab the mushroom caps and heap a plop of filling on all.
4. Place in the fryer basket and top with a little extra cheese.

Nutrition:

- Calories: 285
- Fat: 20.5 g
- Protein: 8.6 g

Jalapeno Cheese Balls

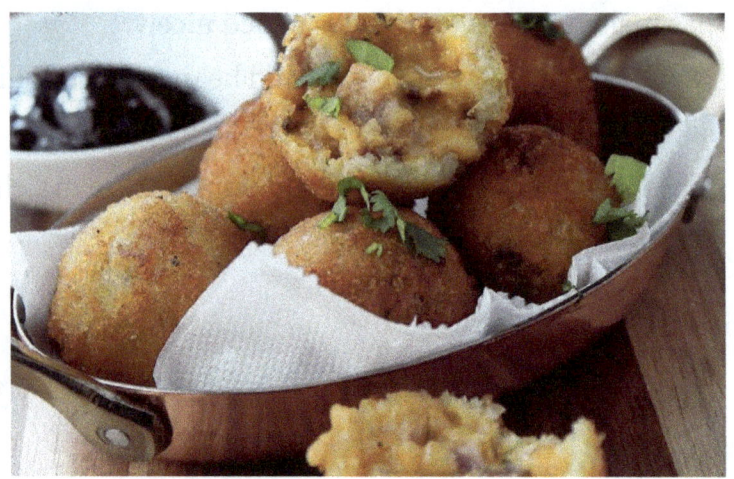

Preparation Time: 10 minutes

Cooking Time: 8 minutes

Servings: 1

Ingredients:

- 1-ounce of cream cheese
- 1/6 cup of shredded mozzarella cheese
- 1/6 cup of shredded Cheddar cheese
- 1/2 jalapeños; finely chopped
- 1/2 cup of breadcrumbs

- 2 eggs
- 1/2 cup of all-purpose flour
- Salt
- Pepper
- Cooking oil

Directions:

1. Mix the cream cheese, mozzarella, Cheddar cheese, and jalapeños in a medium bowl. Mix very well.
2. Form the cheese mixture into balls about an inch thick. You can also use a little ice cream scoop. It works well.
3. Arrange the cheese balls on a sheet pan and place in the freezer for 15 minutes. It can help the cheese balls maintain their shape while frying.
4. Spray the instant Crisp Air Fryer basket with olive oil.
5. Place the breadcrumbs in a small bowl. Beat the eggs in another small bowl. In a third small bowl, mix the flour with salt and pepper to taste, and blend well.
6. Remove the cheese balls from the freezer. Plunge the cheese balls in the flour, then the eggs, then the breadcrumbs.
7. Place the cheese balls in the Instant Crisp Air Fryer. Spray with olive oil. Lock the air fryer lid. Cook for 8 minutes.

8. Open the instant Crisp Air Fryer and flip the cheese balls. I would like to recommend flipping them rather than shaking, so the balls maintain their form. Cook for more 4 minutes.
9. Cool before serving.

Nutrition:
- Calories: 96
- Fat: 6 g
- Protein: 4 g
- Sugar: 0 g

Zucchini Omelet

Preparation Time: 10 minutes

Cooking Time: 10 minutes

Servings: 1

Ingredients:

- 1/2 teaspoon of butter
- 1/2 zucchini; julienned
- 1 egg
- 1/8 teaspoon of fresh basil; chopped
- 1/8 teaspoon of red pepper flakes, crushed
- Salt and newly ground black pepper, to taste

Directions:

1. Preheat the instant Crisp Air Fryer to 355º F.
2. Melt butter on a medium heat using a skillet.
3. Add zucchini and cook for about 3-4 minutes.
4. In a bowl, add the eggs, basil, red pepper flakes, salt, black pepper, and beat well.
5. Add cooked zucchini and gently stir to mix.

6. Transfer the mixture into the instant Crisp Air Fryer pan. Lock the air fryer lid.
7. Cook for about 10 minutes. Also, you might prefer to wait until it is thoroughly done.

Nutrition:

- Calories: 285
- Fat: 20.5 g
- Protein: 8.6 g

Courgette Risotto

Preparation Time: 10 minutes

Cooking Time: 5 minutes

Servings: 8

Ingredients:

- 2 tablespoons of olive oil
- 4 cloves garlic; finely chopped
- 1.5 pounds of Arborio rice
- 6 tomatoes; chopped
- 2 teaspoons of chopped rosemary
- 6 courgettes; finely diced
- 1 ¼ cups of peas; fresh or frozen
- 12 cups of hot vegetable stock
- Salt to taste
- Freshly ground pepper

Directions:

1. Place a large, heavy-bottomed pan over medium heat. Add oil. When the oil is heated, add onion and sauté until translucent.
2. Stir in the tomatoes and cook until soft.
3. Stir in the rice and rosemary. Mix well.
4. Add half the stock and cook until dry. Stir frequently.
5. Add remaining stock and cook for 3-4 minutes.
6. Add courgette and peas and cook until rice becomes soft. Add salt and pepper to taste.
7. Stir in the basil. Let it sit for 5 minutes.

Nutrition:

- Calories: 406
- Fats: 5 g
- Carbohydrates: 82 g
- Proteins: 14 g

Cheesy Cauliflower Fritters

Preparation Time: 10 minutes

Cooking Time: 7 minutes

Servings: 1

Ingredients:

- 1/2 cup of chopped parsley
- 1 cup of Italian breadcrumbs
- 1/3 cup of shredded mozzarella cheese
- 1/3 cup of shredded sharp cheddar cheese
- 1 egg
- 2 minced garlic cloves
- 3 chopped scallions
- 1 head of cauliflower

Directions:

1. Cut the cauliflower up into florets. Wash well and pat dry. Place into a food processor and pulse for 20-30 seconds or till it's like rice.

2. Place the cauliflower rice in a bowl and blend with pepper, salt, egg, cheeses, breadcrumbs, garlic, and scallions.
3. Make 15 patties of the mixture with hands, then add more breadcrumbs if needed.
4. Spritz patties with vegetable oil, and put the fitters into your Instant Crisp Air Fryer. Pile it in a single layer. Lock the air fryer lid. Set temperature to 390°F, and set time to 7 minutes, flipping after 7 minutes.

Nutrition:

- Calories: 209
- Fat: 17 g
- Protein: 6 g
- Sugar: 0.5 g

Bell-Pepper Corn Wrapped in Tortilla

Preparation Time: 5 minutes

Cooking Time: 15 minutes

Servings: 1

Ingredients:

- 1/4 small red bell pepper; chopped
- 1/4 small yellow onion; diced
- 1/4 tablespoon of water
- 1/2 cob of grilled corn kernels
- 1 large tortilla
- One-piece commercial vegan nuggets, chopped
- Mixed greens for garnish

Directions:

1. Preheat the Crisp Air Fryer to 400°F.
2. In a skillet heated over medium heat, sauté the vegan nuggets, onions, bell peppers, and corn kernels. Set aside.
3. Place filling inside the corn tortillas.

4. Lock the air fryer lid. Fold the tortillas and place inside the moment Crisp Air Fryer. Cook for 15 minutes or until the tortilla wraps are crispy.
5. Serve with mixed greens on top.

Nutrition:

- Calories: 548
- Fat: 20.7 g
- Protein: 46 g

Zucchini Parmesan Chips

Preparation Time: 10 minutes

Cooking Time: 8 minutes

Servings: 1

Ingredients:

- 1/2 tsp. of paprika
- 1/2 cup of grated parmesan cheese
- 1/2 cup of Italian breadcrumbs
- 1 lightly beaten egg
- 2 thinly sliced zucchinis

Directions:

1. Use a really sharp knife or mandolin slicer to slice the zucchini as thinly as you can. Pat off extra moisture.
2. Beat the egg with a pinch of pepper, salt, and a bit of water.
3. Combine paprika, cheese, and breadcrumbs in a bowl.
4. Dip slices of zucchini into the egg mixture and then into breadcrumb mixture. Press gently to coat.

5. Mist encrusted zucchini slices with vegetable oil cooking spray. Put them into your Instant Crisp Air Fryer in a single layer. Latch the air fryer lid. Set temperature to 350°F and set time to 8 minutes.
6. Sprinkle with salt and serve with salsa.

Nutrition:

- Calories: 211
- Fat: 16 g
- Protein: 8 g
- Sugar: 0 g

Prosciutto Spinach Salad

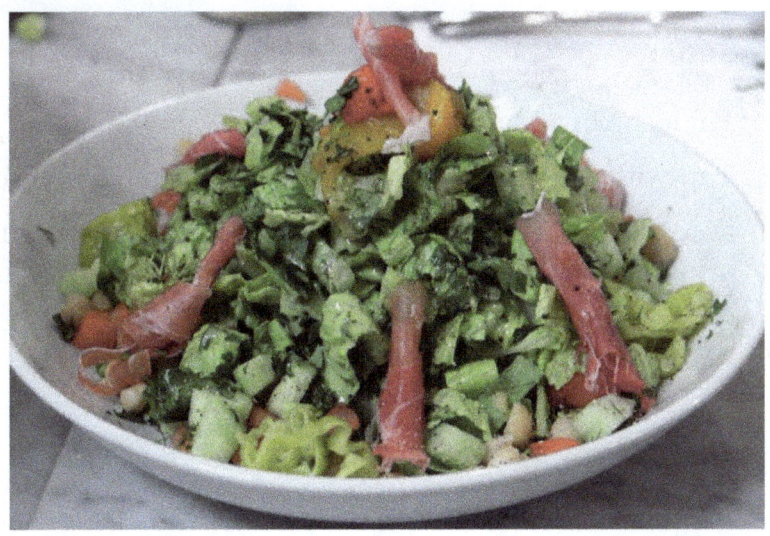

Preparation Time: 5 minutes

Cooking Time: 5 minutes

Servings: 2

Ingredients:

- 2 cups of baby spinach
- 1/3 lb. of prosciutto
- 1 cantaloupe
- 1 avocado
- ¼ cup of diced red onion

- Handful of raw, unsalted walnuts

Directions:

1. Put a cup of spinach on each plate.
2. Top with the diced prosciutto, cubes of melon, slices of avocado, a couple of purple onion, and a couple of walnuts.
3. Add some freshly ground pepper, if you wish.
4. Serve!

Nutrition:

- Calories: 348
- Carbs: 11 g
- Fat: 9 g
- Protein: 26 g
- Fiber: 22 g

Crispy Roasted Broccoli

Preparation Time: 10 minutes

Cooking Time: 8 minutes

Servings: 1

Ingredients:

- 1/4 tsp. of Masala
- 1/2 tsp. of red chili powder
- 1/2 tsp. of salt
- 1/4 tsp. of turmeric powder
- 1 tbsp. of chickpea flour
- 1 tbsp. of yogurt
- 1/2-pound of broccoli

Directions:

1. Cut broccoli up into florets. Immerse in a bowl of water with two teaspoons of salt for at least half an hour to get rid of impurities.
2. Take out broccoli florets from water and allow to drain. Wipe down thoroughly.

3. Mix all other ingredients to make a marinade.
4. Toss broccoli florets into the marinade. Cover and chill for 15-30 minutes.
5. Preheat the instant Crisp Air Fryer to 390° F. Place marinated broccoli florets into the fryer, lock the air fryer lid, set the temperature to 350°F, and set time to 10 minutes. Florets are going to be crispy when done.

Nutrition:

- Calories: 96
- Fat: 1.3 g
- Protein: 7 g
- Sugar: 4.5 g

Grilled Ham & Cheese

Preparation Time: 15 minutes

Cooking Time: 30 minutes

Servings: 2

Ingredients:

- 3 low-carb buns
- 4 slices of medium-cut deli ham
- 1 tbsp. of salted butter
- 1 oz. of flour
- 3 slices of cheddar cheese
- 3 slices of muenster cheese

Directions:

Bread:

1. Preheat your fryer to 350°F/175°C.
2. Mix the flour, salt, and baking powder in a bowl. Set aside.
3. Add in the butter and coconut oil to a skillet.
4. Melt for 20 seconds and pour into another bowl.
5. In this bowl, mix in the dough.

6. Scramble 2 eggs and add to the dough.
7. Add ½ tablespoon of coconut flour to thicken, and place evenly in a cupcake tray. Fill about ¾ inch.
8. Bake for 20 minutes or until browned.
9. Allow to chill for 15 minutes and cut each in half for the buns.

<u>Sandwich:</u>

1. Fry the deli meat in a skillet on a high heat.
2. Put the ham and cheese between the buns.
3. Heat the butter on medium-high.
4. When brown, turn heat to low and add the dough to the pan.
5. Press down with a weight until you smell burning, then flip to crisp each side.
6. Enjoy!

Nutrition:

- Calories: 188
- Carbs: 12 g
- Fat: 16 g
- Protein: 14 g
- Fiber: 18 g

Coconut Battered Cauliflower Bites

Preparation Time: 5 minutes

Cooking Time: 20 minutes

Servings: 1

Ingredients:

- Salt and pepper to taste
- 1 flax egg or 1 tablespoon flaxseed meal + 3 tablespoons of water
- 1 small cauliflower; cut into florets
- 1 teaspoon of mixed spice
- 1/2 teaspoon of mustard powder
- 2 tablespoons of maple syrup
- 1 clove of garlic; minced
- 2 tablespoons of soy sauce
- 1/3 cup of oats flour
- 1/3 cup of plain flour
- 1/3 cup of desiccated coconut

Directions:

1. In a bowl, mix oats, flour, and desiccated coconut. Season with salt and pepper to taste, then set aside.
2. Place the flax egg in another bowl and add a pinch of salt to taste. Set aside.
3. Season the cauliflower with mixed spice and mustard powder.
4. Dredge the florets in the flax egg first, then in the flour mixture.
5. Place it inside the instant Crisp Air Fryer, lock the air fryer lid, and cook at 400°F for 15 minutes.
6. Meanwhile, place the maple syrup, garlic, and soy in a saucepan and heat over medium flame. Wait for it to boil and adjust the heat to low until the sauce thickens.
7. After 15 minutes, remove the florets inside the instant Crisp Air Fryer and place them in the saucepan.
8. Toss to coat the florets, then place them inside the instant Crisp Air Fryer and cook for an additional 5 minutes.

Nutrition:

- Calories: 154
- Fat: 2.3 g
- Protein: 4.69 g

Mashed Garlic Turnips

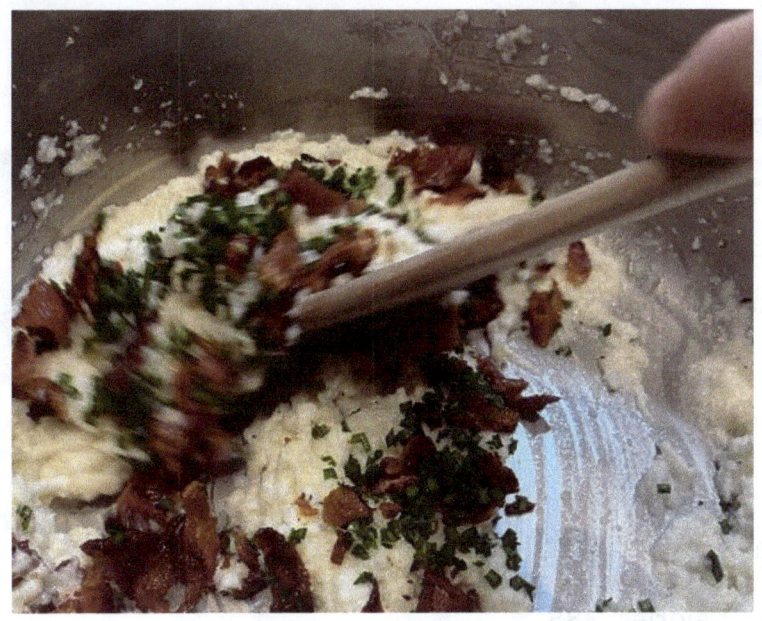

Preparation Time: 5 minutes

Cooking Time: 10 minutes

Servings: 2

Ingredients:

- 3 cups of diced turnip
- 2 cloves of garlic; minced
- ¼ cup of heavy cream

- 3 tbsps. of melted butter
- Salt and pepper to season

Directions:

1. Boil the turnips until it is soft.
2. Drain and mash the turnips.
3. Add the cream, butter, salt, pepper and garlic. Mix very well.
4. Serve!

Nutrition:

- Calories: 488
- Carbs: 32 g
- Fat: 19 g
- Protein: 34 g
- Fiber: 20 g

Air Fryer Asparagus

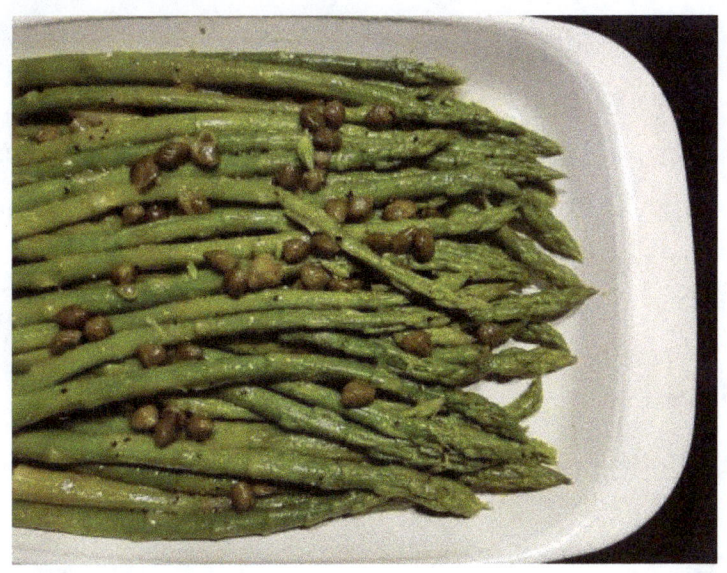

Preparation Time: 5 minutes

Cooking Time: 8 minutes

Servings: 1

Ingredients:

- Nutritional yeast
- Olive oil non-stick spray
- 1 bunch of asparagus

Directions:

1. Wash the asparagus. Don't forget to trim off the thick, woody ends.
2. Spray with olive oil spray and sprinkle with yeast.
3. In your Instant Crisp Air Fryer, lay the asparagus in a singular layer. Set the temperature to 360°F. Set the time to 8 minutes.

Nutrition:

- Calories: 17
- Fat: 4 g
- Protein: 9 g
- Avocado Fries

Diced Cauliflower & Curry Chicken

Preparation Time: 15 minutes

Cooking Time: 30 minutes

Servings: 6

Ingredients:

- 2 lbs. of chicken (4 breasts)
- 1 packet of curry paste
- 3 tbsps. of ghee (can substitute with butter)
- ½ cup of heavy cream
- 1 head of cauliflower (around 1 kg)

Directions:

1. In a large skillet, melt the ghee.
2. Add the curry paste and blend.
3. Once mixed, add a cup of water and simmer for 5 minutes.
4. Add the chicken, cover the skillet and simmer for 18 minutes.
5. Cut a cauliflower head into florets and blend in a food processor to form the diced cauliflower.

6. When the chicken is cooked, uncover, add the cream and cook for more 7 minutes.
7. Serve!

Nutrition:
- Calories: 267
- Carbs: 42 g
- Fat: 31 g
- Protein: 34 g
- Fiber: 32 g

Jalapeno Coins

Preparation Time: 10 minutes

Cooking Time: 5 minutes

Servings: 1

Ingredients:

- 1 egg
- 2/3 tbsp. of coconut flour
- 1 sliced and seeded jalapeno
- Pinch of garlic powder
- Pinch of onion powder
- Bit of Cajun seasoning (optional)
- Pinch of pepper and salt

Directions:

1. Ensure your Instant Crisp Air Fryer is preheated to 400º F.
2. Mix all dry ingredients.
3. Pat jalapeno slices dry. Dip them into the egg wash, and then into the dry mixture. Toss to coat thoroughly.

4. Add coated jalapeno slices to Instant Crisp Air Fryer in a singular layer. Spray with vegetable oil.
5. Lock the air fryer lid. Set temperature to 350°F and set time to 5 minutes. Cook till just crispy.

Nutrition:

- Calories: 128
- Fat: 8 g
- Protein: 7 g
- Sugar: 0 g

Lasagna Spaghetti Squash

Preparation Time: 30 minutes

Cooking Time: 90 minutes

Servings: 6

Ingredients:

- 25 slices of mozzarella cheese
- 1 large jar (40 oz.) of Rao's Marinara sauce
- 30 oz. of whole-milk ricotta cheese
- 2 large spaghetti squash; cooked (44 oz.)
- 4 lbs. of ground beef

Directions:

1. Preheat your fryer to 375°F/190°C.
2. Slice the spaghetti squash and place it face down inside a fryer proof dish. Fill with water until covered.
3. Heat for 45 minutes or until the skin is soft.
4. Roast the meat until it browns.
5. In a large skillet, heat the browned meat and marinara sauce. Put aside when warm.

6. Scrape the flesh off the cooked squash to resemble strands of spaghetti.
7. Layer the lasagna in a large greased pan in alternating layers of spaghetti squash, meat sauce, mozzarella, and ricotta. Repeat until all are layered.
8. Bake for 30 minutes and serve!

Nutrition:

- Calories: 508
- Carbs: 32 g
- Fat: 8 g
- Protein: 22 g
- Fiber: 21 g

Monkey Salad

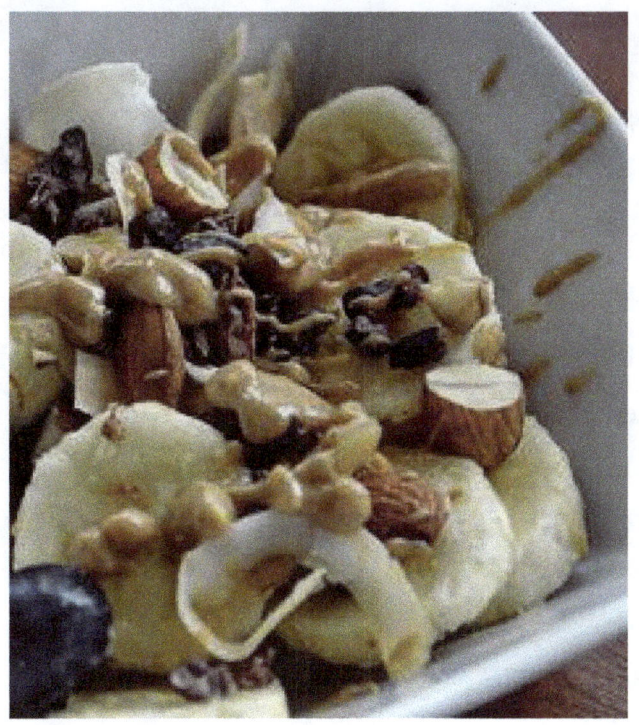

Preparation Time: 4 minutes

Cooking Time: 7 minutes

Servings: 1

Ingredients:

- 2 tbsps. of butter
- 1 cup of unsweetened coconut flakes

- 1 cup of raw, unsalted cashews
- 1 cup of 90% dark chocolate shavings

Directions:

1. In a skillet, melt the butter on a medium heat.
2. Add the coconut flakes and sauté until it becomes lightly browned or for 4 minutes.
3. Add the cashews and sauté for 3 minutes. Remove from the heat and sprinkle with bittersweet chocolate shavings.
4. Serve!

Nutrition:

- Calories: 321
- Carbs: 5 g
- Fat: 12 g
- Protein: 6 g
- Fiber: 5 g

Mu Shu Lunch Pork

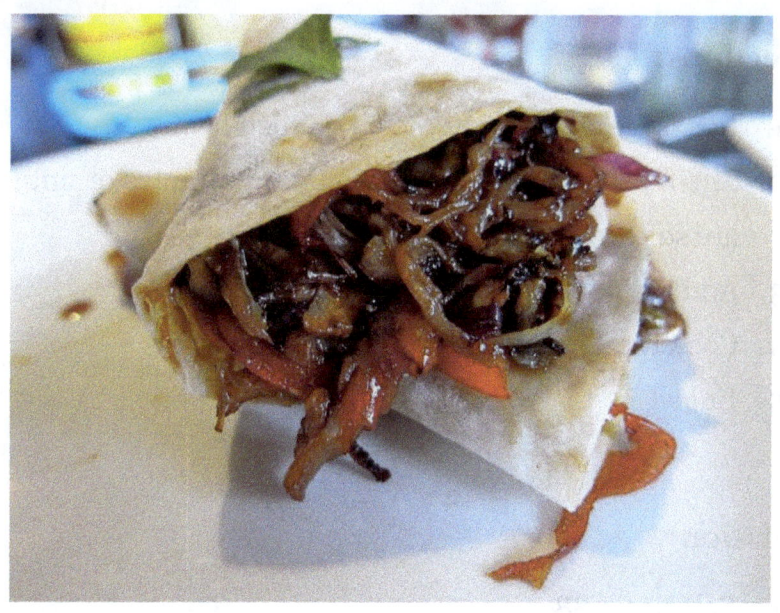

Preparation Time: 5 minutes

Cooking Time: 10 minutes

Servings: 2

Ingredients:

- 4 cups of coleslaw mix, with carrots
- 1 small onion; sliced thin
- 1 lb. of cooked roast pork; cut into ½" cubes
- 2 tbsps. of hoisin sauce

- 2 tbsps. of soy sauce

Directions:

1. In a large skillet, heat the oil on high heat.
2. Stir-fry the cabbage and onion for 4 minutes or until they are soft.
3. Add the pork, hoisin, and soy sauce.
4. Cook until browned.
5. Enjoy!

Nutrition:

- Calories: 388
- Carbs: 16 g
- Fat: 21 g
- Protein: 25 g
- Fiber: 16 g

Fiery Jalapeno Poppers

Preparation Time: 10 minutes

Cooking Time: 40 minutes

Servings: 4

Ingredients:

- 5 oz. of cream cheese
- ¼ cup of mozzarella cheese
- 8 medium jalapeno peppers
- ½ tsp. of Mrs. Dash Table Blend
- 8 slices of bacon

Directions:

1. Preheat your fryer to 400°F/200°C.
2. Cut the jalapenos in half.
3. Use a spoon to scrape out the insides of the peppers.
4. In a bowl, mix together the cream cheese, mozzarella cheese and spices of your choice.
5. Pack the cheese mixture into the jalapenos and place the peppers on top.

6. Wrap each pepper in 1 slice of bacon, from bottom to top.
7. Bake for 30 minutes. Broil for a further 3 minutes.
8. Serve!

Nutrition:

- Calories: 238
- Carbs: 4 g
- Fat: 10 g
- Protein: 24 g
- Fiber: 14 g

Bacon & Chicken Patties

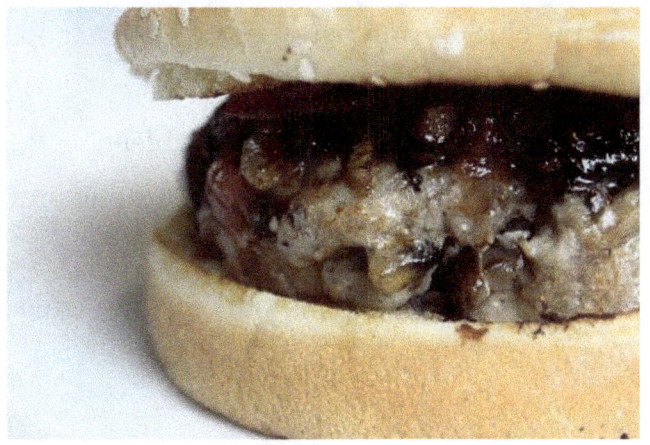

Preparation Time: 5 minutes

Cooking Time: 15 minutes

Servings: 2

Ingredients:

- 1 ½ oz. of can chicken breast
- 4 slices of bacon
- ¼ cup of parmesan cheese
- 1 large egg
- 3 tbsp. of flour

Directions:

1. Cook the bacon until crispy.
2. Blend the chicken and bacon together in a food processor until they become smooth.
3. Add in the parmesan, egg, flour and blend.
4. Make the patties by hand and fry on a medium heat in a pan with some oil.
5. Once browned, flip over, continue cooking, and allow them to drain.
6. Serve!

Nutrition:

- Calories: 387
- Carbs: 13 g
- Fat: 16 g
- Protein: 34 g
- Fiber: 28 g

Garlic Chicken Balls

Preparation Time: 15 minutes

Cooking Time: 10 minutes

Servings: 4

Ingredients:

- 2 cups of ground chicken
- 1 teaspoon of minced garlic
- 1 teaspoon of dried dill
- 1/3 carrot; grated
- 1 egg; beaten
- 1 tablespoon of olive oil
- ¼ cup of coconut flakes
- ½ teaspoon of salt

Directions:

1. Mix together ground chicken, minced garlic, dried dill, carrot, egg, and salt in a bowl.
2. Stir the chicken mixture with your fingertips until it is homogenous.

3. Then make medium balls from the mixture.
4. Coat every chicken ball in coconut flakes.
5. Heat up vegetable oil in the skillet.
6. Add chicken balls and cook them for 3 minutes on all sides. The cooked chicken balls should have a golden-brown color.

Nutrition:

- Calories: 200
- Fat 11.5 g
- Fiber 0.6 g
- Carbs 1.7 g
- Protein 21.9 g

Cheddar Bacon Burst

Preparation Time: 25 minutes

Cooking Time: 90 minutes

Servings: 8

Ingredients:

- 30 slices of bacon
- 2 ½ cups of cheddar cheese
- 4-5 cups of raw spinach
- 1-2 tbsp. of Tones Southwest Chipotle Seasoning
- 2 tsps. of Mrs. Dash Table Seasoning

Directions:

1. Preheat your fryer to 375°F/190°C.
2. Weave the bacon into 15 vertical pieces & 12 horizontal pieces. Cut the additional 3 in half to fill in the rest, horizontally.
3. Season the bacon.
4. Add the cheese to the bacon.
5. Add the spinach and depress to compress.
6. Tightly roll up the woven bacon.

7. Line a baking sheet with kitchen foil and add much salt to it.
8. Put the bacon on top of a cooling rack and put that on top of your baking sheet.
9. Bake for 60-70 minutes.
10. Allow to cool for 10-15 minutes.
11. Slice and enjoy!

Nutrition:

- Calories: 218
- Carbs: 20 g
- Fat: 9 g
- Protein: 21 g
- Fiber: 5 g

Blue Cheese Chicken Wedges

Preparation Time: 20 minutes

Cooking Time: 45 minutes

Servings: 4

Ingredients:

- Blue cheese dressing
- 2 tbsps. of crumbled blue cheese
- 4 strips of bacon
- 2 chicken breasts (boneless)
- 3/4 cup of your favorite buffalo sauce

Directions:

1. Boil a large pot of salted water.
2. Put two chicken breasts into the pot and cook for 28 minutes.
3. Turn off the heat and let the chicken rest for 10 minutes. Using a fork, tear the chicken apart into strips.
4. Cook and cool the bacon strips and then set aside.
5. On a medium heat, mix the chicken and buffalo sauce. Stir until it's hot.

6. Add the bleu and buffalo pulled chicken. Top with the cooked bacon crumble.
7. Serve and enjoy.

Nutrition:
- Calories: 309
- Carbs: 27 g
- Fat: 18 g
- Protein: 34 g
- Fiber: 29 g

www.ingramcontent.com/pod-product-compliance
Lightning Source LLC
Chambersburg PA
CBHW070733030426
42336CB00013B/1961